WORKOUT AND EXERCISE PLANS FOR BEGINNERS.

"Beginner's Guide to Fitness and Easy Bodybuilding Routine for a Healthier You"

Jenny Pearl

Table Of Contents

Introduction

Meet Sam, a regular office worker with a newfound desire for a healthier lifestyle. Like many beginners, Sam stands at the crossroads of fitness, armed with enthusiasm but clueless about where to start. That's where "FitStart: Your Beginner's Handbook for Workout and Exercise Plans" comes into play – a beacon of simplicity in a world of complex fitness advice.

In this book, you won't find complicated jargon or routines that make your head spin. Instead, imagine a friendly guide that holds your hand through the basics, turning fitness from a daunting challenge into an exciting journey. FitStart is more than a book; it's your companion, helping you take those first steps towards a fitter, more energized version of yourself.

The approach is refreshingly straightforward. No need for fancy gym equipment or hours of intense workouts. FitStart embraces simplicity, offering easy-to-follow plans that seamlessly integrate into your daily life. It's not about pushing yourself to the limit; it's about discovering your own pace and enjoying the process.

What makes FitStart stand out is its commitment to understanding your body. Every exercise is explained in plain language, so you're not just going through the motions – you're building a connection with your body. This book isn't about perfection; it's about progress. Whether you're a complete beginner or someone who's dabbled in fitness before, FitStart meets you where you are, guiding you towards a healthier lifestyle with patience and encouragement.

Bid farewell to overwhelming fitness choices and dive into a world where simplicity meets effectiveness. FitStart is more than just a guide; it's a friend cheering you on during every squat, jog, and stretch. You'll discover the joy of movement, the satisfaction of breaking a sweat, and the empowerment that comes with taking charge of your well-being.

So, if you've ever felt lost in the maze of workout advice, fear not. FitStart is here to simplify the journey, making fitness not just accessible but enjoyable. Get ready to transform your routine into a celebration of progress with FitStart – because every small step is a triumph on the path to a healthier, happier you.

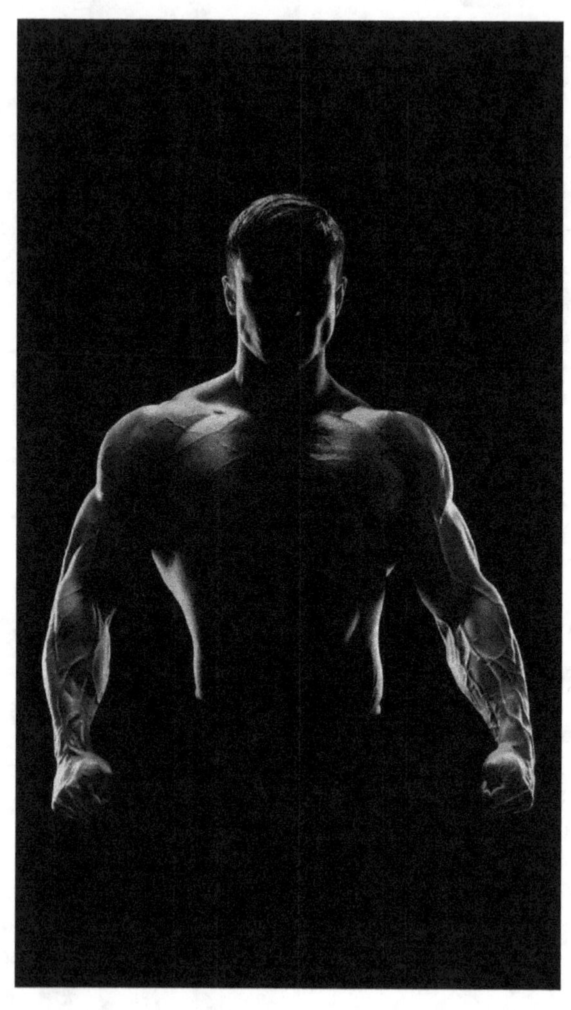

Chapter 1

Start Here: A Beginners Guide

Welcome to "Start Here: A Beginner's Guide," the compass for anyone eager to embark on a transformative journey into the world of fitness. In a realm often clouded by complexity, this book is your friendly navigator, simplifying the path to a healthier, happier you.

Imagine standing at the entrance of a lush forest, the air filled with anticipation. "Start Here" is your guide through the trees, each page unveiling the beauty of exercise in its simplest form. No fitness jargon, no daunting routines—just a clear, easy-to-follow roadmap designed specifically for beginners.

Open the book, and you'll find a colorful array of exercises, each introduced with a warm invitation to dive in. From basic stretches to low-impact workouts, "Start Here" ensures that every step feels like a victory, no matter where you are in your fitness journey.

This isn't about perfection; it's about progress. "Start Here" encourages you to embrace the joy of movement without the pressure of unattainable goals. The focus is on starting, on taking that initial step towards a healthier lifestyle. With simplicity as its guiding principle, this book transforms exercise from a chore into a delightful discovery.

"Start Here" is unique because of its dedication to inclusivity.It doesn't matter if you're a fitness novice or someone starting over; this guide meets you exactly where you are. The exercises are tailored to accommodate various fitness levels, ensuring that everyone can find their comfortable starting point.

As you navigate through these pages, you'll realize that "Start Here" isn't just a guide; it's a companion. It stands beside you, cheering you on as you explore the world of wellness. This book isn't a one-size-fits-all solution; it's an invitation to create a fitness routine that aligns with your uniqueness.

So, whether you're stepping onto the fitness path for the first time or seeking a fresh beginning, let "Start Here" be your go-to guide. Simple, unique, and filled with encouragement, this book promises to make your initial steps into exercise an enjoyable adventure. Welcome to the starting line – your journey begins here.

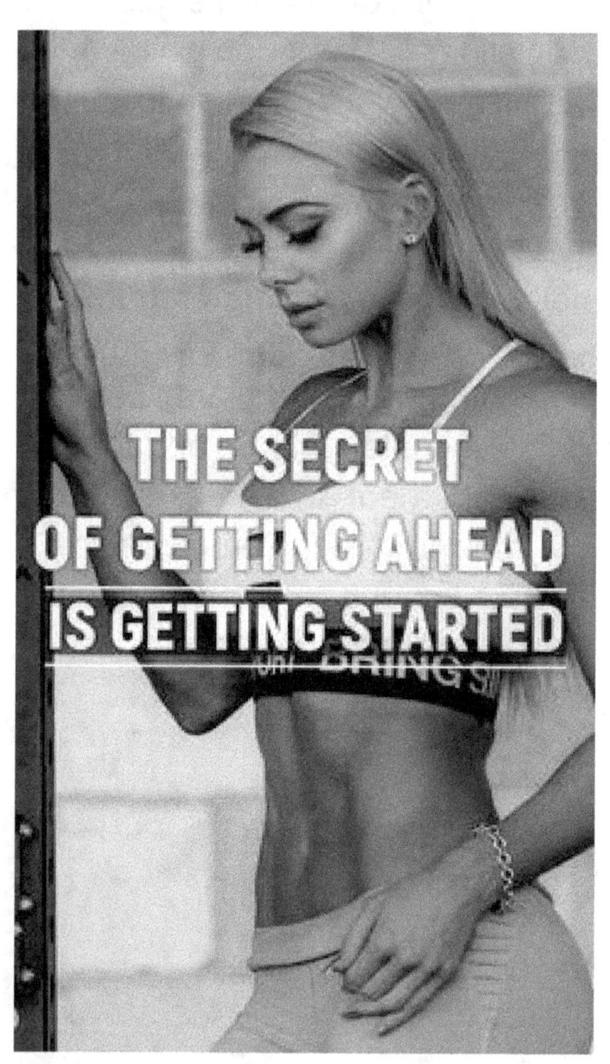
THE SECRET
OF GETTING AHEAD
IS GETTING STARTED

Chapter 2

Know Your Body: Body Basics 101

"Know Your Body: Body Basics 101" is the key that unlocks the door to a healthier, more informed fitness journey. This book is your personal tour guide through the fascinating landscape of your own body, making the complex world of exercise as simple as A, B, C.

Imagine you're embarking on a grand adventure, and your body is the map. "Know Your Body" ensures you understand the terrain before taking your first step. This isn't a lecture; it's a friendly conversation about the incredible machine you inhabit.

Open the pages, and you'll discover colorful illustrations and easy-to-digest explanations. From bones to muscles, the book breaks down the basics, allowing you to appreciate the marvels of your body. No medical jargon here—just simple, relatable insights that make you go, "Ah, so that's how it works!"

But "Know Your Body" doesn't stop at anatomy; it delves into the language your body speaks. It introduces you to signals like fatigue, soreness, and flexibility, helping you understand the subtle cues your body sends. This isn't just about exercise; it's about building a connection with the vessel that carries you through life.

What sets this book apart is its commitment to empowerment. "Know Your Body" isn't about imposing rules; it's about giving you the tools to listen to your body's unique needs. It encourages a partnership where you become the captain of your wellness ship, navigating the seas of fitness with newfound confidence.

As you flip through the pages, you'll see that "Know Your Body" isn't a textbook—it's a user-friendly manual for the incredible adventure of self-discovery. This book aims to make you not just a participant in your fitness journey but an informed, enthusiastic captain steering towards a healthier, happier horizon.

So, whether you're a complete beginner or someone looking to deepen your understanding, "Know Your Body: Body Basics 101" is your passport to a more connected, empowered, and harmonious relationship with your body. Prepare to set out on a journey of wellbeing and self-discovery.

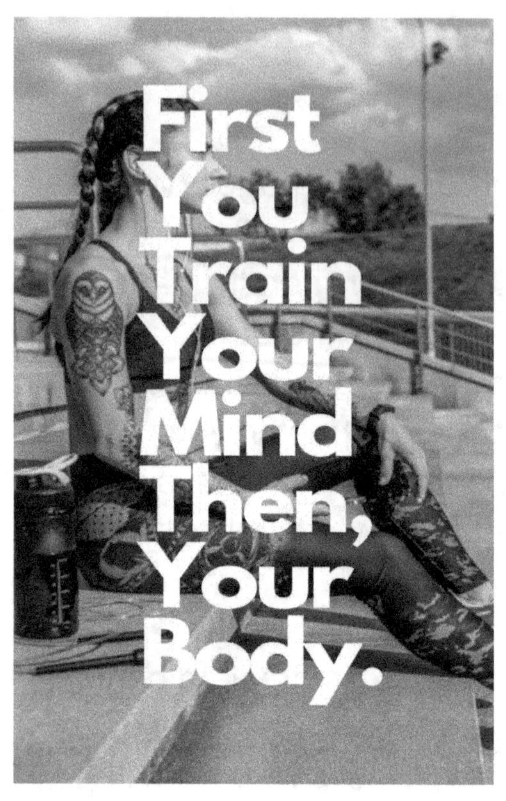
First
You
Train
Your
Mind
Then,
Your
Body.

Chapter 3

Goal Setting For Success

"Goal Setting for Success" in your fitness journey is like plotting stars on a map; it gives your workouts direction and purpose. In this book tailored for beginners, we're not talking about climbing Mount Everest on day one. Instead, think of it as planting seeds – small, achievable goals that blossom into a garden of success.

Picture this: You, the gardener of your fitness dreams, sowing seeds of progress. "Goal Setting for Success" breaks down your aspirations into manageable steps. From mastering a new exercise to increasing stamina, each goal is like a stepping stone, guiding you towards triumph.

What makes this book stand out is its simplicity. No overwhelming resolutions or unrealistic expectations – just clear, bite-sized goals that celebrate your journey. "Goal Setting for Success" encourages you to define your ambitions, making your fitness path a personalized adventure.

Whether it's committing to a certain number of workouts per week or conquering a specific exercise, this book transforms your aspirations into achievable milestones. Remember, success isn't a distant mountain; it's the everyday hills you conquer. With "Goal Setting for Success," you're not just setting goals; you're creating a roadmap to celebrate victories, big and small, on your way to a healthier, happier you. Get ready to plant those seeds and watch your fitness garden flourish.

Chapter 4

Warm-Up Wonders

"Warm-Up Wonders" is the magic spell that transforms your workout routine from mundane to marvelous. In this book crafted especially for beginners, we're unveiling the secrets behind the curtain – the simple, yet powerful, art of warming up.

Imagine your body as a slumbering dragon, waiting to unleash its full potential. "Warm-Up Wonders" is the gentle nudge that awakens the dragon, preparing it for the feats ahead. This isn't just about stretching; it's about unlocking the wonders within your muscles and joints.

Open the book, and you'll discover a world of dynamic warm-up routines, each designed to be as enjoyable as the main act. No more tedious stretches that feel like a chore – "Warm-Up Wonders" introduces you to movements that make your body dance with anticipation. It's not just about preventing injuries; it's about turning the warm-up into a celebration of movement.

What sets this book apart is its playfulness. Forget the notion that warming up is a serious business. "Warm-Up Wonders" encourages you to embrace the joy of preparing your body for action. From light cardio to dynamic stretches, each warm-up routine is a symphony that tunes your body into harmony.

As you delve into the pages, you'll realize that "Warm-Up Wonders" isn't a prelude; it's an essential part of the fitness performance. It's the gateway to a workout experience that feels like a treat rather than a task. This book invites you to be the conductor of your warm-up orchestra, orchestrating the movements that set the stage for a triumphant fitness journey.

So, whether you're a morning workout enthusiast or an evening exercise explorer, "Warm-Up Wonders" is your ticket to a prelude that turns your fitness routine into a masterpiece. Get ready to tap into the magic of warming up and witness the wonders it brings to your journey toward a healthier, happier you.

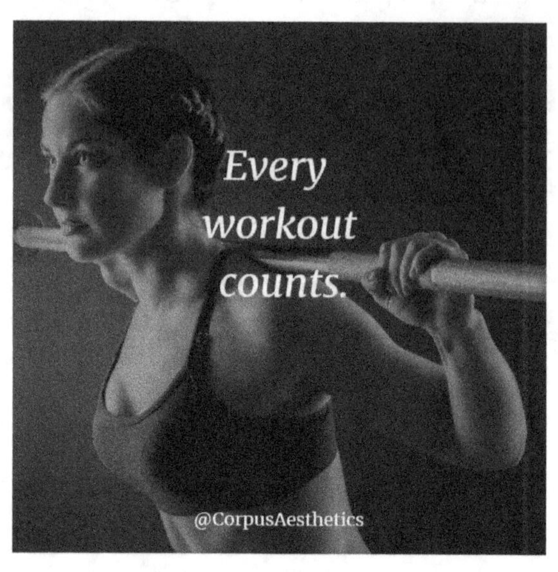
Every
workout
counts.
@CorpusAesthetics

Chapter 5

Cardio Made Simple

"Cardio Made Simple" is your passport to a vibrant, healthier heart in this user-friendly guide for beginners. Imagine cardio not as a daunting task but as a joyful dance – a simple, rhythmic movement that elevates your heart rate and infuses your body with energy.

Open the book, and you'll find a collection of cardio wonders designed to be as straightforward as your favorite dance steps. No need for complex routines or fancy equipment – just uncomplicated, effective exercises that turn cardio into a fun and accessible experience.

What makes "Cardio Made Simple" truly special is its emphasis on enjoyable movement. Say goodbye to tedious treadmill sessions! Instead, embrace exercises that feel like a breath of fresh air, whether it's a brisk walk, a lively dance around your living room, or a playful session of jumping jacks.

This guide is a celebration of variety. "Cardio Made Simple" understands that one size doesn't fit all, offering a diverse range of activities to keep things interesting. It's like having a menu of heart-boosting options, allowing you to choose the cardio adventure that suits your mood and preferences.

As you flip through the pages, you'll discover that this book isn't just about improving cardiovascular health; it's about making cardio a delightful part of your routine. The exercises are carefully crafted to be beginner-friendly, ensuring that whether you're a fitness newbie or returning after a hiatus, you can jump right in.

Get ready to transform cardio from a task into a treat with "Cardio Made Simple." It's time to lace up those metaphorical dancing shoes and discover the joy of heart-healthy movement. This guide isn't just about getting your heart pumping; it's about infusing your fitness journey with simplicity and smiles. Welcome to a world where cardio is not a chore but a celebration of life and vitality.

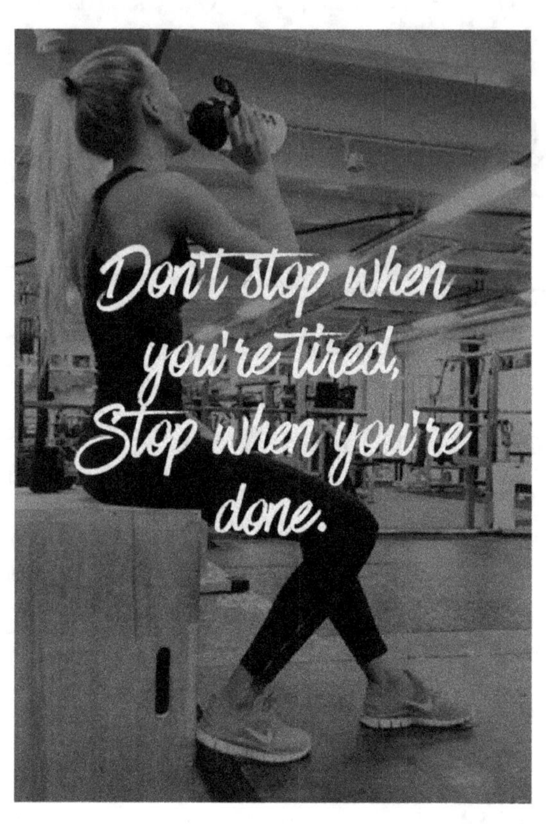
Don't stop when
you're tired,
Stop when you're
done.

Chapter 6

Strength 101: Basic Training

"Strength 101: Basic Training" is your gateway to building a robust foundation in the world of fitness, specially crafted for beginners. Think of strength as the superhero suit your body wears for everyday adventures, and this book is the manual that helps you assemble it, one simple step at a time.

Open the book, and you'll enter a world where strength isn't about lifting gigantic boulders. Instead, it's a gentle introduction to basic exercises that empower you, like the first steps in becoming your own superhero. No need for complicated equipment or confusing terminology – just straightforward, everyday movements that transform you into a stronger version of yourself.

What makes "Strength 101" stand out is its simplicity. It's not about lifting the heaviest weights; it's about understanding the essence of strength and gradually adding layers to your superhero suit. Picture squats, lunges, and push-ups as the fundamental stitches, stitching together the fabric of your newfound strength.

As you embark on your basic training journey, you'll realize that "Strength 101" isn't a boot camp; it's a friendly guide introducing you to your body's incredible capabilities. This book isn't about creating bodybuilders; it's about instilling a sense of confidence and resilience in your everyday life.

So, whether you're a fitness novice or someone ready for a fresh approach, "Strength 101: Basic Training" invites you to pick up your metaphorical superhero cape and start crafting a body that's not just aesthetically pleasing but capable and resilient. Get ready to embrace the simplicity of strength, where each movement becomes a small victory on your journey to becoming your own superhero. Welcome to the beginning of a stronger, more empowered you!

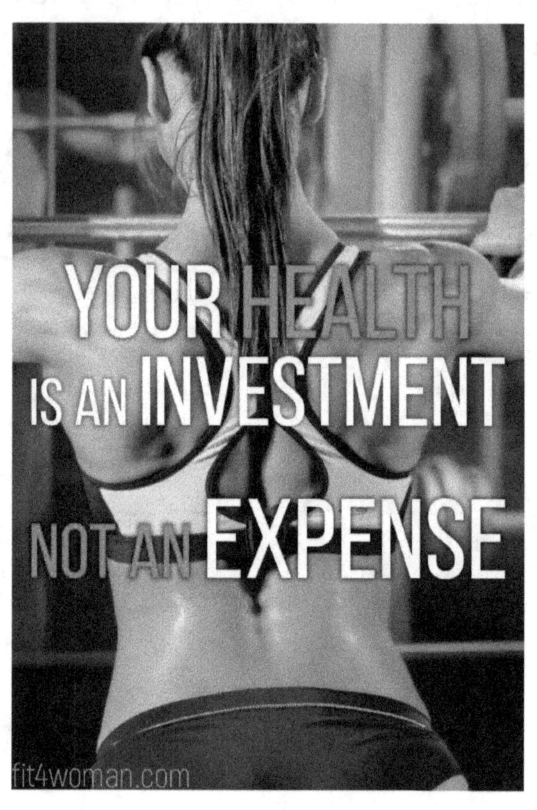

YOUR HEALTH
IS AN INVESTMENT
NOT AN EXPENSE
fit4woman.com

Chapter 7

Flexibility Essentials

"Flexibility Essentials" is like giving your body a gentle stretch, opening the door to a world where mobility meets comfort. Picture your body as a friendly cat, and this book as the soothing purr that guides you through simple stretches, making flexibility accessible and enjoyable for beginners.

As you flip through the pages, you'll find that "Flexibility Essentials" is not about becoming a contortionist. It's a roadmap to help you move with ease, whether you're reaching for something on a high shelf or tying your shoelaces. No need for advanced yoga poses; this book is your gentle introduction to the basics.

What sets this guide apart is its simplicity. "Flexibility Essentials" introduces easy-to-follow stretches that anyone can do, regardless of age or fitness level. Think of it as giving your muscles a spa day – a chance to unwind and become more limber. Each stretch is like a mini-vacation for your body.

The beauty of "Flexibility Essentials" lies in its adaptability. It's not a rigid routine; it's a collection of stretches that can be incorporated into your daily life. Whether you're at home, in the office, or outdoors, these flexibility wonders are designed to seamlessly fit into your routine.

This guide isn't about contorting your body into pretzel shapes; it's about fostering a sense of fluidity and ease. "Flexibility Essentials" is your friendly companion, encouraging you to embrace the joy of movement without stiffness. So, whether you're a beginner looking to touch your toes or someone seeking relief from everyday tension, get ready to discover the essentials of flexibility – because a supple, comfortable body is just a stretch away. Welcome to the world where flexibility isn't a challenge but a delightful journey towards a more mobile and relaxed you.

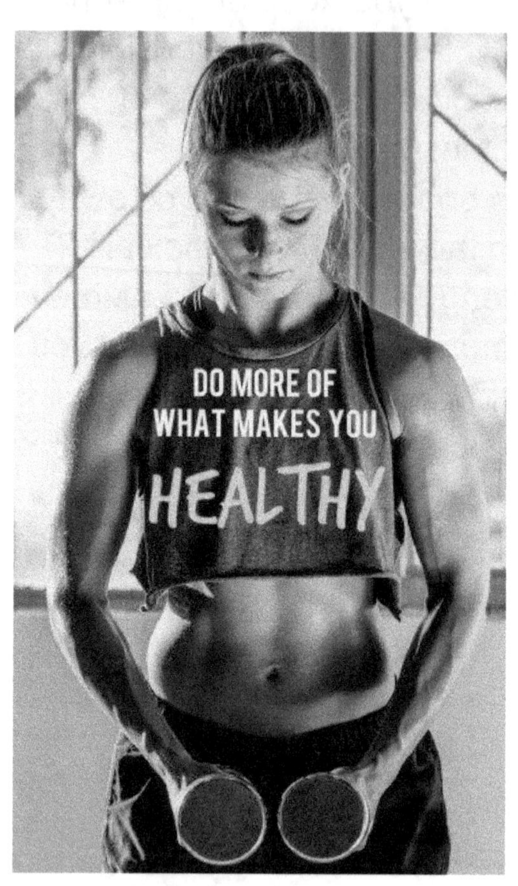

DO MORE OF
WHAT MAKES YOU
HEALTHY

Chapter 8

Core Strength Unleashed

"Core Strength Unleashed" is your guide to unlocking the powerhouse within you, turning your core into a strong and stable foundation. Imagine your core as the superhero of your body, and this book as the secret manual to unleashing its strength, making every movement feel like a confident stride through life.

As you flip through the pages, you'll step into a world where core strength isn't just about six-pack abs; it's about feeling centered, balanced, and ready for anything. "Core Strength Unleashed" simplifies the journey for beginners, offering plain English insights into the essentials of building a resilient and powerful core.

What makes this guide stand out is its straightforward approach. No need for complicated exercises or confusing terminology. "Core Strength Unleashed" introduces you to simple, effective movements that target your core muscles. From basic planks to gentle twists, each exercise is a key to unlocking the potential of your core without overwhelming complexity.

Picture this: Every crunch, every twist, is like turning the key to unleash the superhero within. This book isn't about achieving unattainable feats; it's about creating a strong, supportive core that enhances your daily life. Whether you're picking up groceries or playing with your kids, "Core Strength Unleashed" is your ally, ensuring you do it with confidence and ease.

As you embark on the journey through this guide, you'll discover that core strength isn't just about aesthetics; it's about functional fitness. It's the secret sauce that transforms your body into a well-coordinated, resilient machine. So, whether you're a beginner or someone looking to redefine your core approach, get ready to unleash the strength within. With "Core Strength Unleashed," you're not just building a strong core; you're fostering a foundation that supports you in every step of your journey. Welcome to the world where your core becomes the superhero it was always meant to be—strong, powerful, and ready for action.

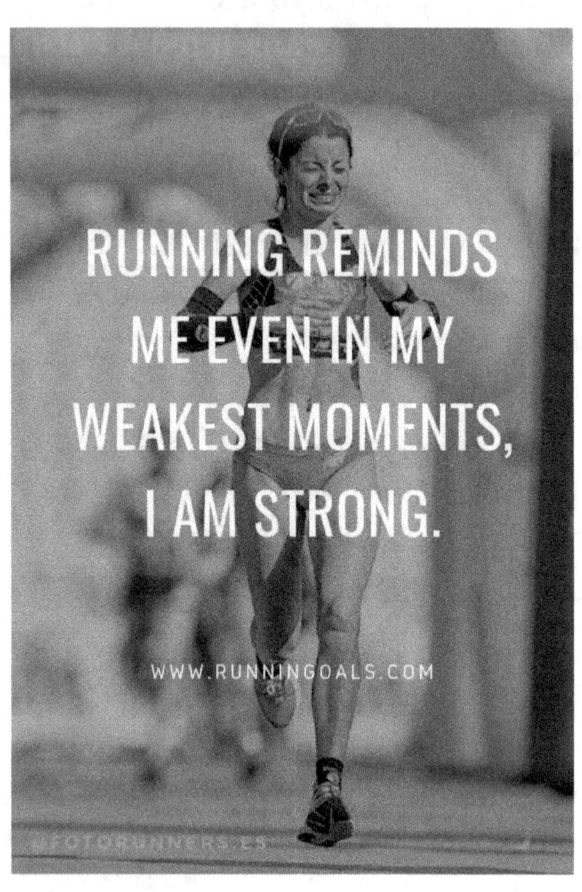
RUNNING REMINDS
ME EVEN IN MY
WEAKEST MOMENTS,
I AM STRONG.
WWW.RUNNINGOALS.COM

Chapter 9

Full-Body Bliss: Beginners Workout

"Full-Body Bliss: Beginners Workout" invites you to a joyful fitness experience where every muscle gets its moment to shine. Picture this as a friendly gathering of your body parts, each excited to join the celebration of movement. This book is your cordial host, introducing you to the basics of a full-body workout with simplicity as its guiding star.

As you open the book, you step into a world where workouts are not a tedious checklist but a delightful sequence of exercises. No need for complicated gym equipment or confusing routines; "Full-Body Bliss" is about embracing straightforward movements that make your entire body dance with joy.

What makes this workout guide truly unique is its plain English approach. It's not about memorizing complex terms or mastering intricate techniques; it's about connecting with your body in a language you both understand. From head to toe, this workout encompasses easy-to-follow exercises that create a symphony of full-body bliss.

As you progress through "Full-Body Bliss," you'll realize that fitness isn't a chore; it's a celebration. The guide gently encourages you to explore the wonders of movement, appreciating the versatility of your body. It's not just about building strength; it's about experiencing the joy of every stretch, squat, and twist.

This isn't a book about high-intensity workouts that leave you exhausted; it's about cultivating a sense of full-body well-being. From warm-up to cool-down, "Full-Body Bliss" is your companion in creating a routine that feels like a gift to your body. So, whether you're a beginner taking the first steps or someone seeking a fresh approach, get ready to experience the bliss of a full-body workout that celebrates every inch of your incredible self. With "Full-Body Bliss," you're not just exercising; you're dancing through a workout that brings happiness to your entire body—one simple move at a time. Welcome to a world where fitness is a delightful celebration of you.

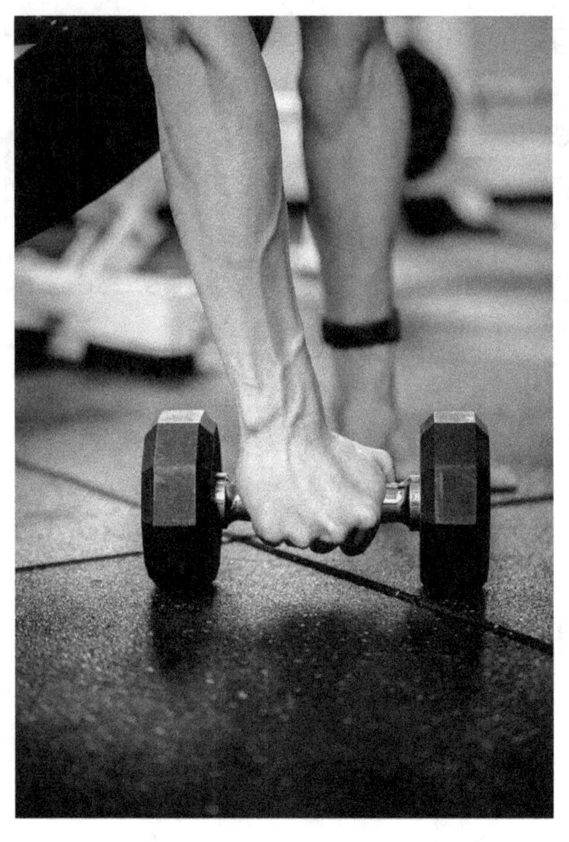

Chapter 10

Resistance Training Demystified

"Resistance Training Demystified" is your friendly guide to unveiling the secrets behind building strength, designed specifically for beginners. Imagine your muscles as eager apprentices, and this book as their mentor, simplifying the art of resistance training into easy-to-understand steps.

Open the book, and you'll enter a world where lifting weights isn't about becoming a bodybuilder overnight. It's a straightforward journey, like adding tools to your body's toolkit. "Resistance Training Demystified" breaks down the barriers for beginners, offering plain

English guidance to sculpt a stronger, more resilient you.

What makes this guide unique is its commitment to simplicity. No need for perplexing techniques or intimidating equipment. "Resistance Training Demystified" introduces you to the basics, making resistance training as simple as lifting, pushing, and pulling. These are the essentials that empower your muscles without complicating the process.

As you explore this book, you'll realize that resistance training isn't just about lifting heavy weights; it's about progressively challenging your muscles. The guide gently encourages you to embrace the learning curve, to understand that every lift is a step towards building functional strength at your own pace.

This isn't a book about extreme workouts; it's about making resistance training accessible. From bodyweight exercises to gradually incorporating resistance, "Resistance Training Demystified" is your mentor in creating a body that feels strong and capable. So, whether you're a beginner taking your first steps into the world of strength or someone seeking a fresh perspective, get ready to demystify resistance training. With "Resistance Training Demystified," you're not just lifting weights; you're building a foundation of strength, one simple lift at a time. Welcome to a world where resistance training is as approachable as adding tools to your fitness toolkit.

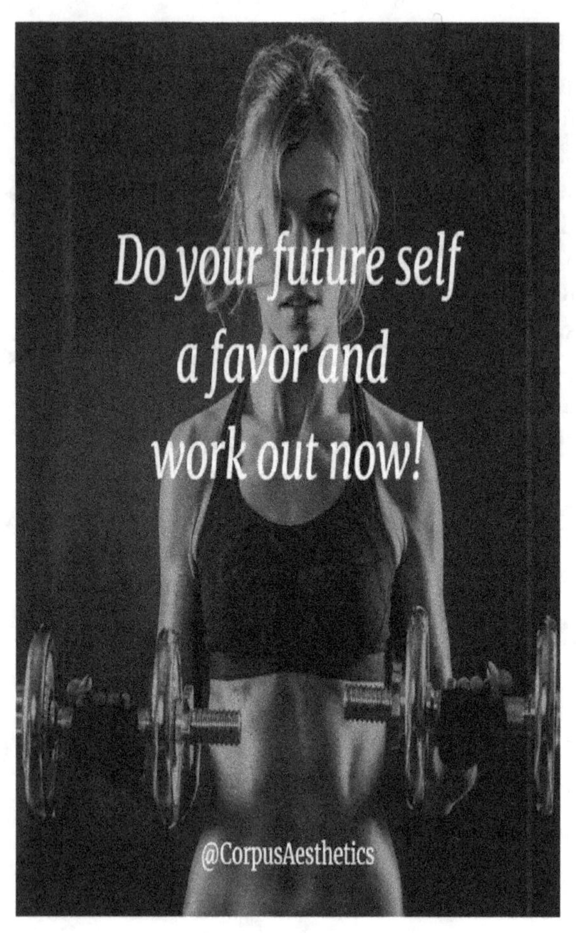

Do your future self
a favor and
work out now!
@CorpusAesthetics

Chapter 11

Endurance For Beginners

"Endurance for Beginners" is your roadmap to a world where stamina isn't a distant mountain but a series of achievable peaks, designed especially for those taking their first steps into the realm of fitness. Imagine your body as a resilient traveler, and this book as the guide offering a simple, clear path toward building enduring strength and vitality.

As you open the book, you step into a space where endurance isn't about exhausting marathons but a series of enjoyable journeys. "Endurance for Beginners" simplifies the fitness adventure, offering plain English insights and a user-friendly plan that transforms the idea of endurance into an accessible and rewarding pursuit.

What sets this guide apart is its commitment to simplicity. No need for daunting long runs or overwhelming intensity. "Endurance for Beginners" introduces you to gradual, effective strategies that make building stamina feel like a friendly exploration. From brisk walks to interval training, these are the essentials that transform the concept of endurance into an achievable and fulfilling goal.

As you follow the guide, you'll discover that endurance isn't just about finishing a race; it's about embracing the joy of sustained movement. The book gently encourages you to find your pace, celebrate progress, and view endurance as a journey rather than a destination.

This isn't a book about extreme challenges; it's about making endurance training approachable and enjoyable. "Endurance for Beginners" is your companion on the path to a more enduring, energized you. So, whether you're starting from scratch or seeking a fresh perspective on stamina building, get ready to explore the world of endurance in a way that feels simple, achievable, and uniquely yours. With this guide, you're not just building endurance; you're embarking on a fulfilling journey towards a more resilient, energetic you—one steady step at a time. Welcome to a world where endurance becomes a joyful and accessible pursuit.

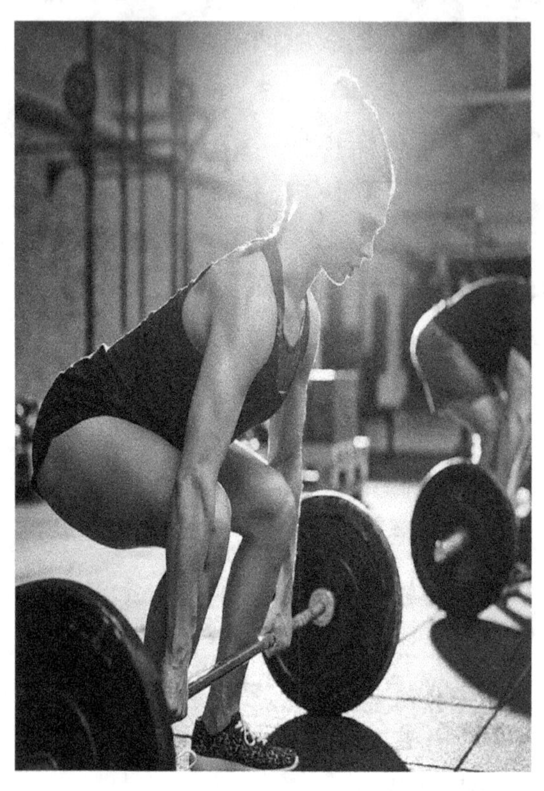

Chapter 12

Your Personalized Workout Plan

"Your Personalized Workout Plan" is like having a fitness roadmap made just for you – tailored to your preferences, pace, and lifestyle. Imagine your fitness journey as a unique story, and this book as your storyteller, simplifying the art of creating a workout plan that aligns with your individual needs.

As you flip through the pages, you're stepping into a realm where fitness isn't one-size-fits-all; it's about celebrating your uniqueness. "Your Personalized Workout Plan" demystifies the complexities, offering a plain English guide to craft a routine that fits seamlessly into your life.

What sets this book apart is its
commitment to simplicity. No need for
rigid routines or overwhelming
exercises. "Your Personalized Workout
Plan" empowers you to choose activities
you enjoy, making your fitness journey a
positive experience. From brisk walks to
dancing in your living room, these are
the essentials that turn your workout
plan into a source of joy.

As you navigate through the book, you'll
realize that your personalized plan isn't
about following someone else's routine;
it's about creating a sustainable,
enjoyable habit that suits your pace. The
guide gently encourages you to listen to
your body, embrace variety, and
progress at a rhythm that feels right for
you.

This isn't a book about strict rules; it's
about making fitness flexible and fun.
"Your Personalized Workout Plan" is

your ally in designing a routine that aligns with your goals and preferences, turning exercise into a positive and personalized adventure. So, whether you're a complete beginner or someone looking for a fresh start, get ready to embark on a fitness journey that's uniquely yours. With this guide, you're not just following a workout plan; you're writing your own story of well-being—one simple choice at a time. Welcome to a world where your workout plan is as unique as you are.

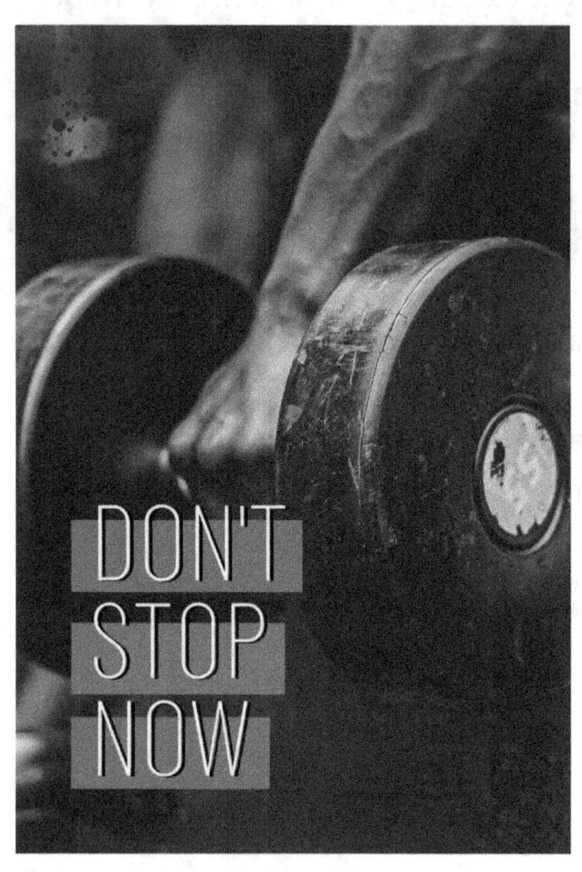

DON'T
STOP
NOW

Chapter 13

Balancing Cardio And Strength

"Balancing Cardio and Strength" is like creating a delicious recipe for your fitness routine, where cardio and strength are the perfect ingredients. Imagine your workout as a well-prepared meal, and this book as your friendly chef, simplifying the process of combining cardio and strength for beginners.

Open the book, and you step into a world where workouts aren't either/or but a harmonious blend. "Balancing Cardio and Strength" embraces simplicity, offering plain English guidance to help you create a routine that's both heart-pumping and muscle-boosting.

What makes this guide unique is its commitment to balance. No need for complicated equations or exhaustive schedules. "Balancing Cardio and Strength" introduces you to easy, effective exercises that incorporate both elements seamlessly. From brisk walks to bodyweight exercises, these are the essentials that turn your routine into a balanced fitness feast.

As you navigate through the book, you'll realize that balancing cardio and strength isn't about choosing sides; it's about enjoying the benefits of both. The guide encourages you to find your rhythm, understand the role of each component, and create a routine that feels satisfying and well-rounded.

This isn't a book about conflicting workouts; it's about creating a balanced fitness plate that caters to your goals and preferences. "Balancing Cardio and Strength" is your partner in designing a routine that combines the heart-healthy benefits of cardio with the muscle-building advantages of strength training. Whether you're a beginner or someone seeking a fresh approach, get ready to embrace the synergy of cardio and strength. With this guide, you're not just exercising; you're crafting a balanced and enjoyable fitness experience—one simple, well-blended move at a time. Welcome to a world where your workout routine is a perfect fusion of cardio and strength, creating a balanced and fulfilling journey.

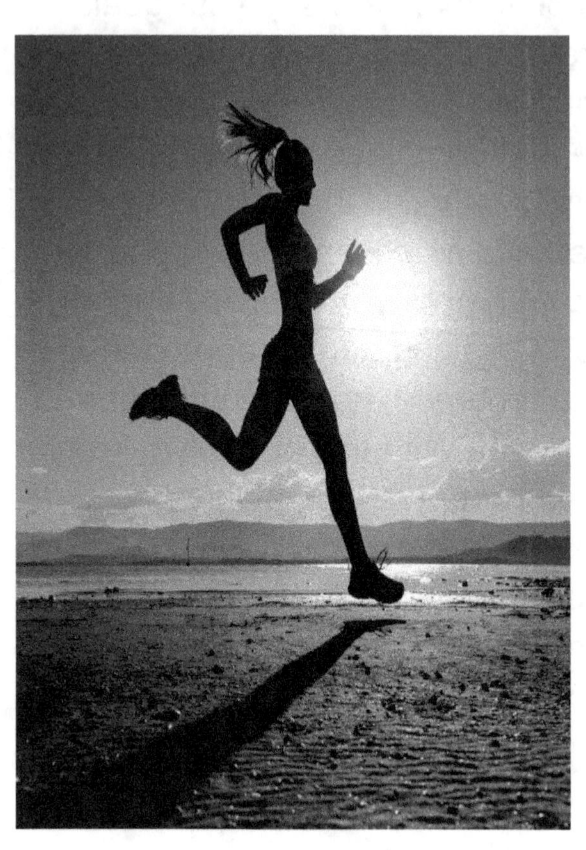

Chapter 14

Rest And Recovery 101

"Rest and Recovery: Your Body's Recharge" is like granting your muscles a well-deserved vacation – an essential chapter in the book of fitness for beginners. Imagine your body as a superhero needing a power nap, and this book as the guide, simplifying the importance of rest and recovery in your exercise journey.

Open the book, and you'll step into a world where rest isn't just a pause but a crucial part of your workout routine. "Rest and Recovery" is all about simplicity, offering plain English wisdom to beginners, highlighting the magic that happens when your body takes a break.

What makes this guide unique is its commitment to the rejuvenating power of rest. No need for complicated schedules or guilt about taking a day off. "Rest and Recovery" introduces you to the simplicity of allowing your body to recharge. From a good night's sleep to rest days between workouts, these are the essentials that transform your exercise routine into a sustainable and enjoyable journey.

As you navigate through the book, you'll realize that rest isn't a sign of weakness; it's a secret weapon for progress. The guide gently encourages you to listen to your body, to understand the language of fatigue, and to embrace the rejuvenating effects of rest.

This isn't a book about pushing through exhaustion; it's about honoring your body's need for recovery. "Rest and Recovery" is your partner in crafting a workout plan that includes ample downtime, making exercise a long-term, joyful experience. So, whether you're a beginner or someone looking to appreciate the importance of rest, get ready to embrace the art of recovery. With this guide, you're not just resting; you're giving your body the gift of renewal—one simple, rejuvenating break at a time. Welcome to a world where rest is a vital ingredient, ensuring your fitness journey is not just active but also balanced and sustainable.

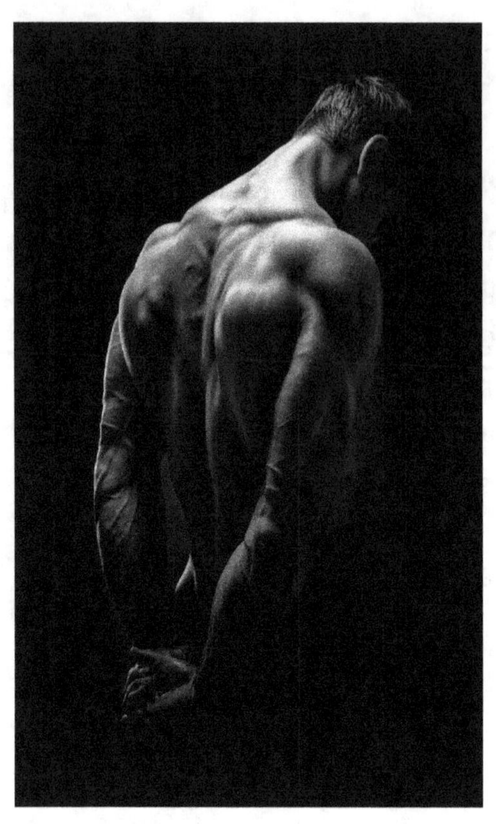

Chapter 15

Stay Motivated Throughout

"Stay Motivated Throughout" is your friendly coach in the grand fitness marathon, ensuring that your enthusiasm stays sprinting alongside you from the starting line to the finish tape. Picture your motivation as a trusty running buddy, and this book as the cheering crowd, offering plain English guidance to keep your spirits high throughout the entire workout and exercise journey.

As you embark on this guide, imagine it as a roadmap filled with colorful signposts to guide you through the terrain of motivation. "Stay Motivated Throughout" is all about simplicity, providing straightforward strategies for beginners, making sure motivation becomes a constant companion rather than an occasional visitor.

What sets this guide apart is its commitment to making motivation an effortless part of your routine. No need for convoluted techniques or intense interventions. "Stay Motivated Throughout" introduces you to practical and enjoyable methods to sustain your enthusiasm. From celebrating small victories to finding joy in the process, these are the essentials that transform motivation from a fleeting feeling into a steady, uplifting force.

As you flip through the pages, you'll discover that staying motivated isn't a mysterious art; it's about cultivating a positive mindset. The guide gently encourages you to embrace the journey, to appreciate progress, and to find joy in the process rather than fixating on the end goal.

This isn't a book about forcing motivation; it's about creating an environment where enthusiasm naturally thrives. "Stay Motivated Throughout" is your partner in crafting a sustainable and enjoyable fitness experience. Whether you're a beginner setting foot on the track or someone seeking a fresh approach, get ready to embrace the art of staying motivated.

With this guide, you're not just following a workout plan; you're weaving motivation into the fabric of your fitness routine—one simple, motivating moment at a time. Welcome to a world where enthusiasm is not just a starting point but a constant companion, making your exercise journey a joyous, uplifting adventure from the first step to the final stretch.

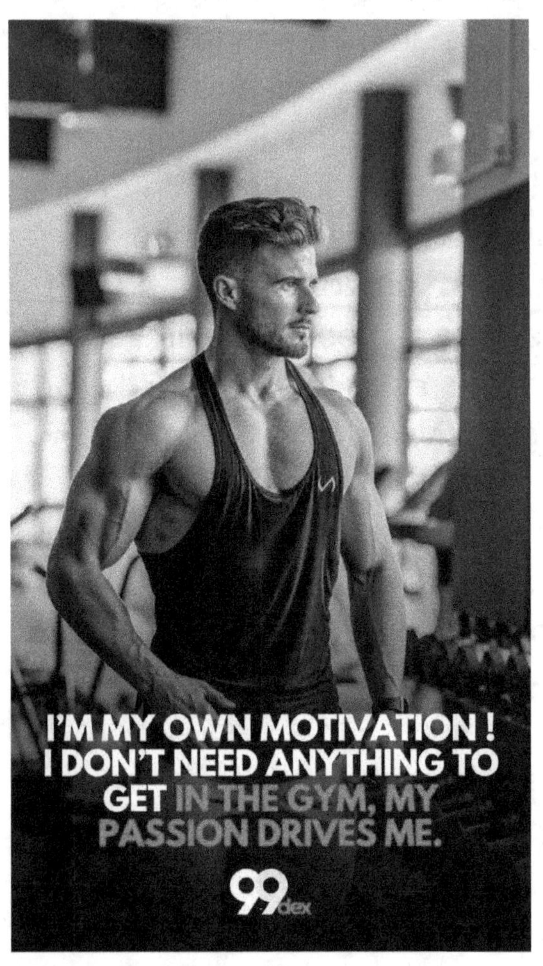
I'M MY OWN MOTIVATION !
I DON'T NEED ANYTHING TO
GET IN THE GYM, MY
PASSION DRIVES ME.
99dex

Chapter 16

Beginners Guide To Nutrition

"Beginner's Guide to Nutrition" is your roadmap to the fuel that powers your fitness journey, designed especially for newcomers to the world of exercise. Imagine your body as a high-performance car, and this book as the manual, simplifying the essentials of nutrition in plain English to ensure your engine runs smoothly throughout your workout and exercise plans.

Open the book, and you step into a world where nutrition isn't a complex science but a straightforward strategy to support your wellness. "Beginner's Guide to Nutrition" demystifies the language, offering plain English guidance to beginners, making the path to a balanced and nourishing diet accessible.

What makes this guide stand out is its commitment to simplicity. No need for calorie counting or complicated meal plans. "Beginner's Guide to Nutrition" introduces you to easy, effective principles that transform your approach to food. From understanding macronutrients to making informed food choices, these are the essentials that make nutrition a friendly companion in your fitness journey.

As you explore the chapters, you'll realize that nutrition isn't about strict diets; it's about building a sustainable relationship with food. The guide gently encourages you to view meals as opportunities to nourish your body, to appreciate the role of hydration, and to cultivate habits that align with your well-being.

This isn't a book about restrictions; it's about making informed choices that suit your lifestyle. "Beginner's Guide to Nutrition" is your partner in creating a balanced and enjoyable eating routine, making nutrition an integral and straightforward aspect of your fitness adventure. So, whether you're a beginner or someone looking to refine your approach, get ready to embrace the world of nutrition with clarity. With this guide, you're not just eating; you're nourishing your body with a simple and effective nutrition plan—one delicious, balanced bite at a time. Welcome to a world where nutrition is not a complicated puzzle but a key ingredient in your journey to a healthier, happier you.

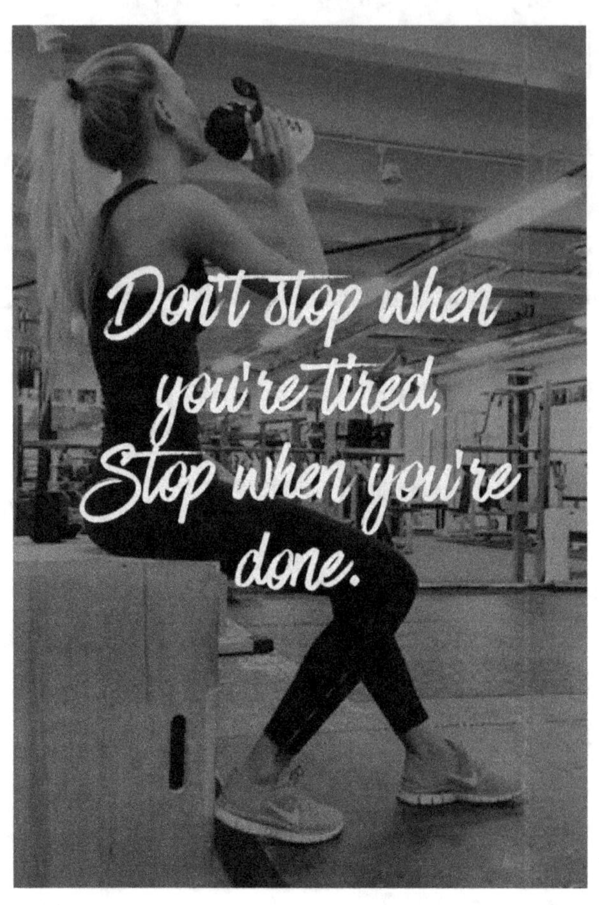
Don't stop when
you're tired,
Stop when you're
done.

Chapter 17

Stay Hydrated

Staying hydrated is a crucial aspect of any successful workout and exercise plan, especially for beginners embarking on their fitness journey. Water is like the superhero of your body – it keeps everything running smoothly and ensures you get the most out of your workouts.

When you exercise, you sweat, and that's your body's way of cooling down. But with each drop of sweat, you lose water. Think of it as your body's natural air conditioner, and water is the coolant. If you don't replenish the lost fluids, it's like running your air conditioner without adding more coolant – things can get overheated.

So, here's the deal: drink water before, during, and after your workout. It's like fueling up your car before a long drive and making sure it has enough gas to keep going. Before you start exercising, sip on some water to hydrate your body. During your workout, take small sips whenever you feel thirsty. And after you've crushed that workout, celebrate with another round of water.

Now, let's talk about signs that your body might be thirsty. It's like your body sending out an SOS signal. Feeling thirsty is an obvious one – it's like your body waving a flag saying, "Hey, I need water!" But there are sneakier signals too, like feeling tired, dizzy, or having a headache. That's your body's way of saying, "I'm low on coolant, help me out!"

Make it a habit to carry a water bottle with you wherever you go, especially when you're exercising. It's like having your trusty sidekick on hand, ready to save the day. And here's a little tip: if your pee looks like lemonade, you're on the right track. If it's more like apple juice, well, it's time to up your water game.

Remember, staying hydrated isn't just for the gym – it's a 24/7 job. Your body is like a plant, and water is its sunlight. So, whether you're sweating it out during a workout or chilling on the couch, keep that water flowing. It's the secret sauce to feeling awesome, energized, and ready to tackle whatever your workout plan throws at you. So, bottoms up, my fitness friend!

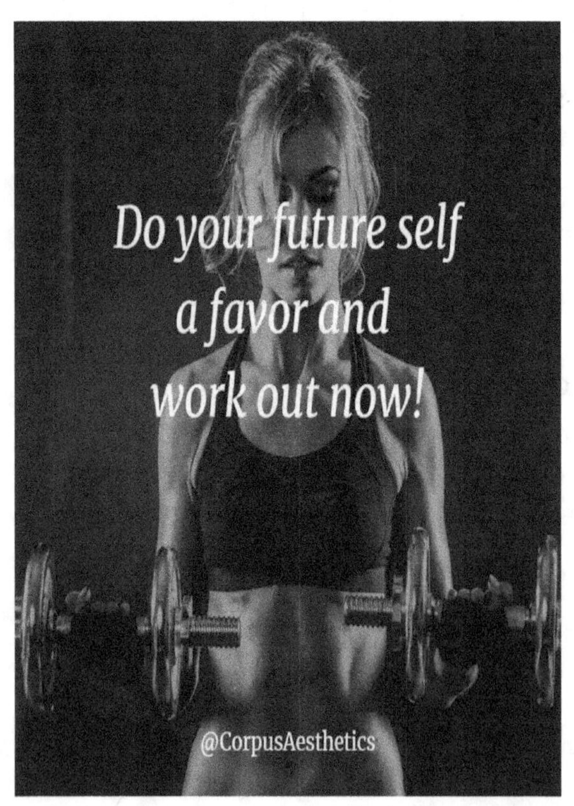

Do your future self
a favor and
work out now!
@CorpusAesthetics

Chapter 18

The Sleep-Fitness Connect

Ah, sleep – the unsung hero of your fitness journey! If your workouts are like the superhero training montage, then sleep is the crucial scene where the hero recharges. Let's break it down in plain English for all you beginners out there.

Imagine your body as a busy workshop. When you exercise, you create little repair jobs for your muscles. Guess what happens when you sleep? Your body goes into superhero mode, fixing those muscles and making them stronger. It's like having a team of handy workers making upgrades while you're catching those Zs.

Now, let's talk about energy – your body's fuel. Lack of sleep is like running on an empty tank. Your workouts might feel like trying to drive a car with no gas – not very effective. When you're well-rested, your energy levels are sky-high, and you're ready to tackle those lunges and push-ups like a fitness warrior.

Oh, and here's the scoop on cravings and willpower. Ever notice how it's harder to resist that tempting snack when you're tired? Blame it on the sleep-deprived gremlins messing with your willpower. When you get enough shut-eye, you're better equipped to say no to those sneaky cravings and stick to your fitness plan.

Think of sleep as the VIP pass to the muscle-building party. It's during those sweet dreams that your body releases growth hormone, helping your muscles grow and repair. So, if you want those biceps to pop and those abs to show, make sure you're catching those Zs like a pro.

In a nutshell, sleep isn't just downtime – it's prime time for your body to work its magic. It's the secret sauce that makes your workouts more effective and keeps you on track with your fitness goals. So, put on those comfy pajamas, tuck yourself in, and let your body do the heavy lifting while you dream of your fitness victories. Sweet dreams, fitness champs!

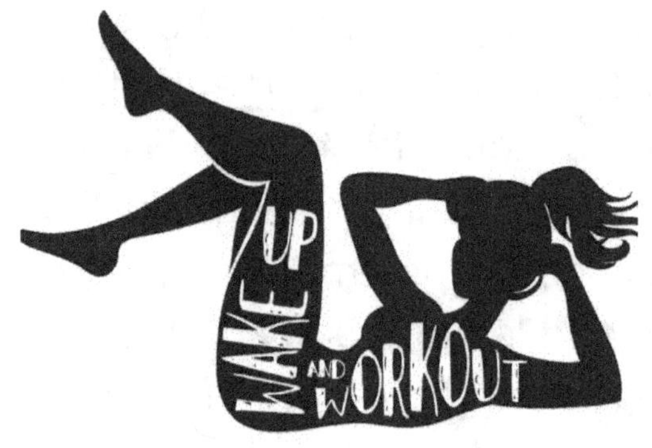

GET HEALTHY U

Chapter 19

Track Your Progress

Tracking your progress is like having a map for your fitness adventure – it helps you see where you've been and where you're headed. Imagine you're on a treasure hunt, and each workout is a step closer to finding that fitness gold. Here's why keeping tabs on your journey is a game-changer for beginners.

First things first, get yourself a fitness journal or use an app – it's like your trusty treasure map. Write down what exercises you did, how many reps, and how heavy those weights were. It's not about showing off; it's about celebrating the small victories. Maybe last week you struggled with five push-ups, and now you can conquer ten – that's progress worth cheering for!

Now, let's talk about the mirror – your personal reflection of triumph. As you keep at it, you'll notice changes in your body. Maybe those jeans feel a bit looser, or you catch a glimpse of muscles where there weren't any before. That's your body saying, "Hey, I'm getting stronger!" Take note of these victories because they're like the hidden gems on your fitness map.

Tracking your progress is also a great motivator. When you see how far you've come, it's like a boost of energy to keep going. It's like looking back at a steep hill you've climbed and realizing, "Wow, I did that!" Plus, it helps you set new goals – the 'X' marks the spot for your next fitness treasure.

Remember, your fitness journey is unique, like your own special adventure story. Tracking your progress is the key to turning each page and discovering the incredible feats your body is capable of. So, grab your fitness map, document those victories, and enjoy the thrill of watching your own fitness saga unfold. Happy tracking, fitness explorer!

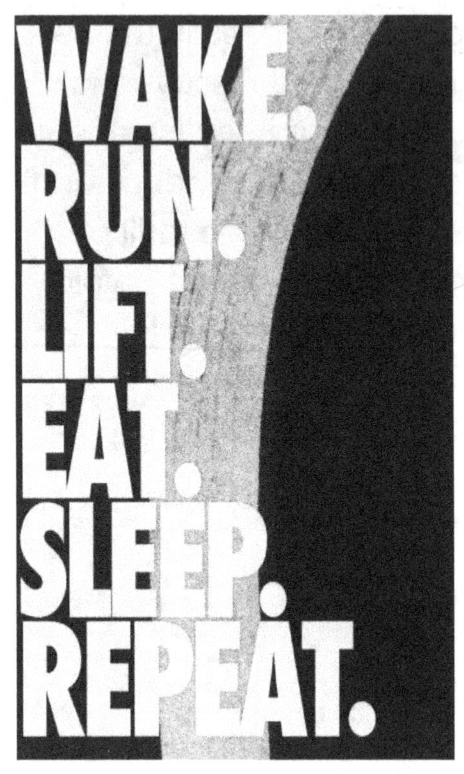

WAKE.
RUN.
LIFT.
EAT.
SLEEP.
REPEAT.

Chapter 20

Overcoming Common Hurdles

Embarking on a workout journey is like setting sail on a fitness adventure. Yet, just like any journey, you might encounter some hurdles along the way. Fear not, brave beginner! Let's navigate through these common obstacles together and keep your fitness ship sailing smoothly.

1. The Time Crunch Conundrum:

"I don't have time!" We've all been there. Life gets busy, and finding time for a workout seems like trying to catch a shooting star. But here's the secret: you don't need hours. Start small – even 15 minutes of exercise can make a difference. It's like planting a seed that grows into a mighty fitness tree.

2. The Motivation Mystery:

"I'm just not feeling it today." Motivation can be as elusive as a hidden treasure. The trick is to make your workouts enjoyable. Find an activity you love – it could be dancing, hiking, or even playing a sport. Turning exercise into something fun is like turning a chore into a treasure hunt. Suddenly, you're excited to dig for gold!

3. The Equipment Enigma:

"I don't have fancy gear." Good news – you don't need a gym full of shiny machines. Your body is a fantastic workout tool. Simple exercises like squats, push-ups, and lunges are like the pirate's toolkit for building strength. No need for a treasure chest of equipment – just use what you have!

4. The Consistency Challenge:

"I keep falling off the wagon." Staying consistent is like navigating stormy seas. The key is not to aim for perfection. Life happens, and that's okay. Treat your fitness journey like a ship – it may sway in the waves, but it keeps moving forward. If you miss a workout, don't abandon ship. Jump back on when the sea is calmer.

5. The Comparison Trap:

"I'm not as fit as others." Comparing yourself to fitness gurus is like comparing your ship to a sleek yacht. Each vessel has its journey. Celebrate your progress, no matter how small. It's like discovering unique treasures on your ship – they may not be gold, but they're invaluable.

6. The Soreness Struggle:

"I ache all over!" Welcome to the land of muscle soreness – a sign you're doing great! Think of it as the aftermath of a thrilling battle. Embrace it, rest when needed, and remember, sore muscles are like battle scars – proof that you're on a victorious fitness quest.

In the grand tale of fitness for beginners, hurdles are merely plot twists. Face them with determination, adapt your course when necessary, and remember: your journey is unlike anyone else's. Overcoming these hurdles is your own unique adventure, full of victories waiting to be discovered. So, hoist the sails and let the fitness odyssey begin!

Chapter 21

Fitness FAQs: Your Questions Answered

Embarking on a fitness journey is like stepping into a world of questions, but fear not – answers are here to guide you through the maze of workout wonderings. Let's tackle some common fitness FAQs, unraveling the mysteries of exercise for beginners.

1. Q: How often should I work out?

Ans: Think of workouts like watering a plant – regular attention is key. Aim for at least 3 to 4 times a week. Start

slow, and gradually increase as your fitness blooms.

2. Q: What's the best time to exercise?

Ans: It's like choosing the perfect playlist – whatever fits your rhythm! Some love mornings for a fresh start, while others prefer evenings to shake off the day's stress. Listen to your body's beat.

3. Q: Do I need fancy equipment?

 Ans: Nope, simplicity rocks! Your body is a powerhouse. Bodyweight exercises like squats, lunges, and push-ups are treasure troves of fitness gold. Equipment is a bonus, not a necessity.

4. Q: How long should my workouts be?

Ans: Quality over quantity! Start with 20-30 minutes and gradually add time. It's like baking – the right ingredients matter more than the baking time.

5. Q: Can I eat before a workout?

Ans: Absolutely! It's like fueling up before a road trip. Choose something light and balanced, like a banana or yogurt. Your body needs energy for the adventure ahead.

6. Q: Is it normal to feel sore after exercising?
Ans: Totally normal! It's like a badge of honor for your hard work. Embrace the muscle soreness – it means you're leveling up. Rest, hydrate, and enjoy the feeling of getting stronger.

7. Q: How do I stay motivated?

Ans: Imagine motivation as your workout playlist – keep it fresh! Set realistic goals, mix up your routines, and celebrate small victories. It's like having a party for your fitness wins.

8. Q: Can I work out if I have health issues?

Ans: Safety first! Consult your doctor and share your fitness plans. Like a customized playlist, they'll help you choose exercises that suit your health tune.

9. Q: What if I miss a workout?

Ans: Life happens – it's okay! Think of it like a rainy day during your beach vacation. Adjust, adapt, and jump back into your routine. Consistency, not perfection, is the goal.

10. Q: How do I know if I'm doing exercises correctly?

Ans: Form is your fitness GPS. Watch tutorials, ask for guidance, or use mirrors. It's like following a recipe – proper form ensures you're cooking up success, not accidents.

In the realm of fitness FAQs, knowledge is your compass. Don't be afraid to ask, explore, and enjoy the adventure. Your fitness journey is a unique story, and these answers are the plot twists that keep you moving forward. Now, let the workout tales begin!

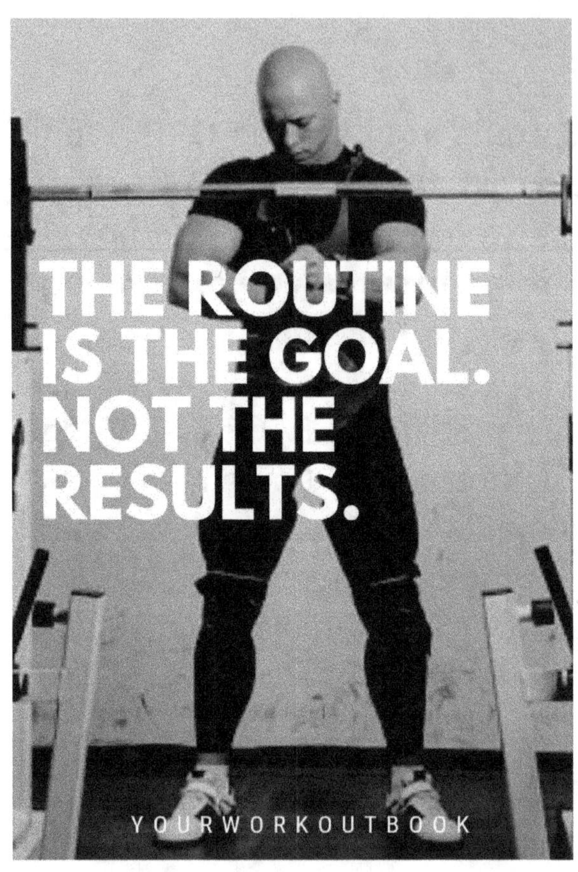
THE ROUTINE
IS THE GOAL.
NOT THE
RESULTS.
YOURWORKOUTBOOK

Chapter 22

Bonus Tips For Quick Results

Fast-track your fitness journey with these bonus tips – the secret sauce for quick results without the overwhelm. Consider these your shortcut to success, fitness enthusiast!

1. Mix It Up Like a Smoothie:

Just like a tasty smoothie blends different ingredients, blend various workouts. It's like giving your muscles a surprise party – they won't get bored, and you'll see quicker progress.

2. HIIT the Ground Running:

High-Intensity Interval Training (HIIT) is like the express train to fitness. Short bursts of intense effort followed by rest periods – it's efficient and burns calories long after your workout is done. Quick and effective – like a fitness ninja move.

3. Snack Smart, Not Hard:

Think of your meals as fuel stations on your fitness highway. Opt for nutritious snacks like fruits, nuts, or yogurt. It's like choosing the premium fuel that keeps your engine running smoothly.

4. Sleep, Your Silent Superpower:

A good night's sleep is like hitting the reset button for your body. It helps muscles recover, boosts energy, and keeps cravings at bay. It's like letting your body charge up for the next day's adventure.

5. Water, the Elixir of Fitness:

Sip, sip, hooray! Water is like your fitness fairy godmother. Drink plenty of it to stay hydrated – it aids digestion, supports your workouts, and keeps you feeling fresh. It's like your own magical potion for success.

6. Celebrate Mini Milestones:

Every step forward is a victory, no matter how small. It's like collecting gold coins on your fitness journey. Celebrate completing a new workout or reaching a personal best – it keeps you motivated and excited for what's next.

7. Buddy System Activated:

Having a workout buddy is like having a personal cheerleader. They keep you accountable, make workouts more fun, and provide that extra push when needed. It's like having a sidekick in your quest for fitness glory.

8. Rest Is Not a Four-Letter Word:

Rest days are like mini-vacations for your muscles. They need time to recover and grow stronger. It's like giving your body a spa day – essential for long-term fitness success.

Incorporate these bonus tips into your fitness routine, and you'll be cruising on the express lane to quick results. Remember, it's not about the destination; it's about enjoying the journey and celebrating every step you take towards a healthier, fitter you. Happy sweating!

Conclusion

Wrapping Up Your Fitness Journey

As you reach the final chapter of your workout and exercise plans for beginners, it's time to reflect, celebrate, and look ahead. Consider this conclusion as the victory lap of your fitness journey – a moment to savor the progress and set the stage for what's to come.

1. Celebrate Small Wins:

Think of your fitness journey as a series of victories, each workout a triumph, and every healthy choice a step forward. Celebrate the small wins – maybe you ran an extra minute, lifted a heavier weight, or simply showed up consistently. It's like collecting medals along the way; every one of them adds to your success story.

2. Reflect on Your Growth:

Take a moment to reflect on where you started and where you are now. It's like looking at before-and-after pictures, not just of your body but of your mindset, energy levels, and overall well-being. Your journey is unique, and every step has contributed to your growth.

3. Embrace the Journey, Not Just the Destination:

Fitness isn't a one-stop destination; it's an ongoing adventure. It's like a road trip where the joy lies in the journey itself. Enjoy the process, savor the workouts, and relish the feeling of becoming a healthier, stronger version of yourself.

4. Set New Goals:

Just as you reached milestones, it's time to set new goals. Think of them as the next chapter of your fitness story. Whether it's running a longer distance, mastering a new exercise, or improving flexibility, your goals are like road signs guiding you to exciting destinations.

5. Listen to Your Body:

Your body is like a wise friend – it communicates its needs. Pay attention to how you feel during and after workouts. If you need rest, take it. If you crave a new challenge, go for it. Listening to your body is like having a reliable GPS on your fitness journey.

6. Share Your Success:

Your journey is inspiring, not just to yourself but to others. Share your successes, big and small. It's like passing the torch of motivation. You might be someone else's inspiration to start their own fitness adventure.

7. Make it a Lifestyle:

Fitness isn't a temporary fix; it's a lifelong commitment. It's like adopting a healthy lifestyle that becomes second nature. Keep making choices that nourish your body, mind, and soul. It's not about perfection but consistency in making positive choices.

As you wrap up this book and the initial phase of your fitness journey, remember that this is just the beginning. Your story continues, filled with more victories, challenges, and moments of growth. Whether you're a beginner or a seasoned fitness enthusiast, the journey is ongoing – embrace it, enjoy it, and keep moving forward. Cheers to a healthier, happier you!.

www.ingramcontent.com/pod-product-compliance
Lightning Source LLC
Chambersburg PA
CBHW070747250726
48662CB00004B/1679